YOUR KNOWLEDGE HAS VALUE

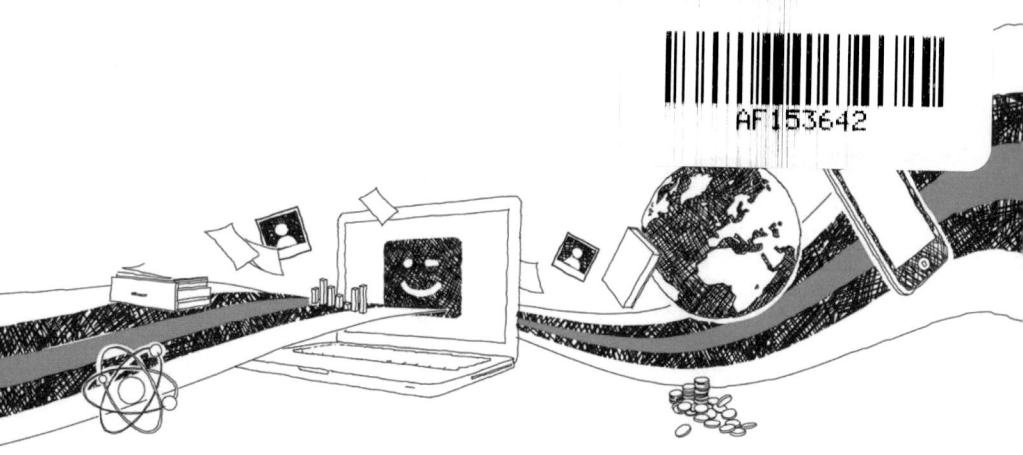
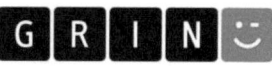

Lewinsohn's Behavioural Theory of Depression. Revolutionary, yet Overgeneralising

Marie-Louise Meiser

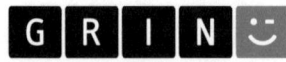

Bibliographic information published by the German National Library:

The German National Library lists this publication in the National Bibliography; detailed bibliographic data are available on the Internet at http://dnb.dnb.de.

ISBN: 9783346426888
This book is also available as an ebook.

© GRIN Publishing GmbH
Nymphenburger Straße 86
80636 München

Print and binding: Books on Demand GmbH, Norderstedt, Germany
Printed on acid-free paper from responsible sources.

The present work has been carefully prepared. Nevertheless, authors and publishers do not incur liability for the correctness of information, notes, links and advice as well as any printing errors.

GRIN web shop: https://www.grin.com/document/1026090

Lewinsohn's Behavioural Theory of Depression: Revolutionary, yet Overgeneralising

Psychology of Mental Health (Conversion), MSc
University of Edinburgh
Word count: 2194

Depression – also known as clinical depression or major depressive disorder (American Psychiatric Association, 2013) – is the most common mental health problem, globally affecting around 300 million people of all ages (World Health Organisation, 2020). It is variable in its causes and presentations, characterised by multivariate symptom complexes – overt behaviour, cognition and somatic symptoms – and an extensive range of functioning (Rehm, 2015). Its comorbidity with various anxiety disorders (Hirschfeld, 2001), behavioural disorders (Daviss & Bond, 2016), and different physical illnesses (Kang et al., 2015) contributes to the disorder's complexity. This symptomatic and antecedent heterogeneity of depression has only partially been considered by behaviourists. Skinner – 'the father of behaviourism' - described depression as an "overt behaviour rather than [a] core affective experience, in line with an operant rather than respondent model" (Kanter et al., 2008, p. 4). This notion became the baseline of Lewinsohn's (1974a) theory of depression which dominated behaviourist literature for a number of decades (Kanter et al., 2008).

According to Lewinsohn's theory, depression is caused by a low, or lack of *response-contingent positive reinforcement*, meaning that insufficient reinforcement causes a reduction of behaviours as well as dysphoria which characterise the main symptoms of depression (Lewinson and Graf, 1973). There are three hypotheses about how a lack of reinforcement arises: Firstly, the environment does not provide sufficient reinforcement; secondly, the individual does not obtain the necessary social skills to receive reinforcement in an environment in which it is actually available; and thirdly, even though the individual obtains reinforcement, they are unable to enjoy it (Abreu & Santos, 2008).When one of these antecedents arises, maladaptive behaviours follow, which themselves lead to lack or loss of positive reinforcement or receiving negative reinforcement. The antecedents, the problem behaviours, and the consequences make up the units of the *three-term contingency* (Skinner, 1953), which interact with each other in a self-perpetuating cycle, also called *chaining* (Rehm,

2015); causing and maintaining depression (Segrin, 2000). In order to evaluate Lewinsohn's theory of depression, his three hypotheses will be examined by drawing from empirical research studies and alternative psychological theories. It is proposed that Lewinsohn's early behavioural theory was revolutionary for our understanding of the aetiology and symptomology of depression, but overgeneralises the heterogeneity of the disorder.

Lewinsohn's Theory: A Revolutionary Approach to the Understanding of Depression

In the following, we will critically examine the extent to which Lewinsohn's theory acted as a revolutionary contribution to our understanding of depression, and whether Lewinsohn's three hypotheses align with recent empirical research studies.

Lewinsohn's hypothesis of the environment not providing sufficient reinforcement contributed to our understanding of reactive depression. Rehm (2015) proposed the example of the loss of a job that once served as a positive reinforcer. Indeed, it has been found that both extrinsic and intrinsic reinforcement is positively linked to employees' impression of doing meaningful work, which in turn has been found to be significantly correlated with employees' well-being (Fairlie, 2013). Supporting this hypothesis, Andreeva et al. (2015) found job loss to consistently predict subsequent depression in both sexes, confirming the outcomes of various other studies on the matter (Bubonya, Cobb-Clark, & Wooden, 2016; Stolove, Galatzer-Levy & Bonanno, 2017; Navarro-Abal et al., 2018). Nevertheless, the self-reported nature of Andreeva et al.'s (2015) data might have caused method and response biases. Furthermore, there was no control for confounding factors, leading to difficulty in establishing a causal link between job loss and depression. It therefore is unclear whether the lack of reinforcement or other variables - such a financial hardship (=social causation hypothesis) - caused depression when experiencing job loss. Nevertheless, due to the vast number of studies indicating one's job has the potential to serve as a positive reinforcer while job loss leads to depression, we can assume that the lack of reinforcement is one factor that leads to depression when facing unemployment. Hence, Lewinsohn's approach was revolutionary for our understanding of lack of reinforcement being an antecedent "of depression with clear environmental precipitants" (Kanter et al., 2008, p.5).

Lewinsohn's model also shed light on cases of chronic depression, where an individual experiences "persistently insufficient levels of reinforcement and social skills deficits that prevent the individual from changing the situation" (Kanter et al., 2008, p.5). According to Lewinsohn (1974), individuals with poor social skills have difficulties receiving positive reinforcement from their environment, and experience punishing events from others leading to and maintaining depression. Supporting this hypothesis, Fauziyyah and Ampuni (2018) found "that lower social skills were associated with higher loneliness and in turn contributed to increasing tendency towards depression" (p. 98), and that depression was correlated with the maintenance of loneliness. These findings are supported by Coyne's (1976) interpersonal theory of depression which posits that individuals' behaviour can elicit social rejection leading to depression and depressive behaviours that maintain social rejection. While Fauziyyah's and Ampuni's (2018) study shows sampling bias due to non-random sampling of college students in a specific cultural context (Indonesia) with gender imbalance (27,91% male, 72,09% female), the vast number of other study outcomes from a variety of samples showing that social skills deficits significantly predict depression (Segrin, 1993, 1996; Cole, Martin, Powers, & Truglio, 1996), and depression significantly predicts social skills deficits (Natale, 1977a, Natale, 1977b) support Lewinsohn's hypothesis. Hence, this hypothesis contributed to our understanding of how social skills deficits can cause depression and maintain it due to the process of *chaining*.

Lewinsohn's hypothesis of depression being caused by a lack of ability to enjoy available reinforcement is based on the idea that social anxiety interferes with the reinforcement, and therefore precedes depression (Lewinsohn, 1974b). Indeed, Schneier et al., (1992) found that social phobia preceded the onset of depression in 69% of their participants, consistent with previous research (Stein et al., 2001). Rodebaugh et al. (2014) discovered that social anxiety leads individuals to report worse friendship quality compared to friend-reports indicating that socially anxious individuals experience less enjoyment from social interactions than their non socially anxious friends. These findings are however limited due to the reliance on self-reports that measured global friendship rather than single friendships. Ratings of specific friendships might have allowed for clearer referents, minimising the possibility of negative attentional biases causing socially anxious participants to focus on less satisfying friendships (Li, Tan & Liu, 2008). Nevertheless, a number of other studies elaborating that characteristic symptoms of social anxiety – such as low self-esteem (Harris & Orth, 2019), negative self-image (Makkar & Grisham, 2011), and underestimation of one's social performance (Stopa, Brown & Hirsch, 2012) – negatively interfere with the enjoyment normally gained from social relationships, supporting Lewinsohn's hypothesis.

Lewinsohn's Theory: An Overgeneralisation of Depression

Although Lewinsohn's theory highlights important factors which cause and maintain depression, it fails to explain the complexity of its aetiology and symptomatology. In the following, we will critically examine the extent to which his three hypotheses overgeneralise depression, and whether the aetiologies and symptoms of depression can be explained by other theories.

Lewinsohn's hypothesis regarding depression arising due to insufficient environmental reinforcement is "based on an implicit assumption that a basic minimum ratio of reinforcement to behaviour is required to maintain an adequate level of functioning" (Rehm, 2015, p. 18). While studies show that an increase of engagement in positively-reinforced events results in positive moods in adolescents, the level of autonomy and personal choice in these activities demonstrated to be mediating factors between the two variables (Weinstein & Mermelstein, 2007). This aligns with the self-determination theory (Deci & Ryan, 1985), asserting that "situational factors that satisfy the basic psychological need of autonomy, namely the perception of one's activities as self-chosen and important, enhance emotional well-being" (Weinstein & Mermelstein, 2007, p. 10). Thus, a simple lack of social activity does not sufficiently explain the development of depression. The factors that contribute to each activity, such as certain associated emotions, might be important variables.

While Lewinsohn's environmental reinforcement hypothesis applies to some cases of reactive depression, it cannot explain endogenous, none-stimulus-bound depression (Kanter et al., 2008). Costello (1972) argues that not only the loss of reinforcers, but the loss of reinforcer effectiveness causes depression, which can be based on endogenous, neurophysiological changes. Although Costello's (1972) hypothesis lacks reliability and validity as it is solely based on observations of depressed individuals, various empirical research studies on biological theories support his hypothesis. It has, for instance, been found that age-related alterations of the endocrine system (Clarke & Currie, 2009) and heightened amygdala response to stress caused by genetic predisposition can trigger depression (Dean & Keshavan, 2017). Nevertheless, one's interaction with "the social environment may influence the development and activity of neural systems, which in turn have an impact on behavioural, physiological, and emotional responses" (Bernaras, Jaureguizar, & Garaigordobil, 2019, p.5).

6

As demonstrated before, lack of social skills can negatively influence interaction with the social environment (Lewinsohn and Graf, 1973). While this hypothesis is broadly supported, a smaller number of studies "with strong methodological features such as a longitudinal design and structured clinical interviews have not supported the model that social skills deficits are antecedents of depression" (Hames, Hagan & Joiner, 2013). Eberhart and Hammen (2006), for instance, neither found actual nor perceived interpersonal problem-solving skills to predict an onset of depression; however, interpersonal problem-solving skills are only one of many behavioural indicators of behavioural skills (Segrin, 2000). Moreover, Eberhart and Hammen's (2006) study was restricted to young women, limiting applicability to other age or gender groups. Interpersonal problem-solving skills were studied as a homogenous construct failing to determine which aspects of interpersonal problem-solving might or might not influence depression. However, as these outcomes are aligned with other longitudinal studies (Wierzbicki, 1984; Wierzbicki & McGabe, 1988), the mixed results raise the question to what extent social skills deficit and depression are actually correlated with one another.

"The disparate findings in this literature may be in part due to differences in the operationalisation of social skills and the levels of depression of the participants across studies" (Hames, Hagan & Joiner, 2013, p.358), which Lewinsohn's theory does not consider: Firstly, the multitude of definitions for 'social skills' raise the question whether researchers are investigating the same concept. Secondly, there are numerous potential moderators of the relationship between social skills and depression: social skills deficits might be more predictive of relapsing into depression rather than causing a first onset thereof (Segrin, 2000); furthermore, social skills deficits might play a different role in primary depression than in secondary depression where "the mechanisms by which poor social skills contribute to depression might be inoperative (or potentially hyperactive) in cases of depression that are secondary to other problems" (Segrin, 2000, p. 396). Thirdly, as depression is significantly

7

associated with reductions in motivation (Beck et al. 2011), it is unclear whether social skills deficits are an individual's incapacity to act in a manner that is considered to be socially appropriate and effective, or whether the individual lacks the motivation to act that way (Segrin, 2000). "This points to the obvious conclusion that the relationship between depression and social skills is multiformed" (Segrin, 2000, p. 396), and that Lewinsohn's theory of the lack of social skills causing and maintaining depression is too simplistic to do this complex relationship justice.

Looking at Lewinsohn's third hypothesis, while social anxiety demonstrated to precede depression (Stein et al., 2001), and lead to the inability to enjoy positively-reinforced social events, this notion overgeneralises the reasons for this inability. Beck's Cognitive Theory of Depression presents an alternative (1967). According to Beck's cognitive triad, "depression is caused by particular stresses that evoke the activation of a schema that screens and codes the depressed individual's experience in a negative fashion" (Ingram, 1984, p. 443), with this distortion of reality being reflected in three areas: oneself, the future and the world (Beck, Epstein & Harrison, 1983). However, the evidential support on this relationship has only been carried out with adolescents (Jabobs & Joseph, 1997), and adults (Pössel, 2009). When testing this on children, 'view of self' and 'view of the future' also significantly predicted depression, but 'view of the world' did not. This might be due to their lack of abstract thinking and therefore not yet having created a world view to the same extent as adults have (Braet et al., 2015). Thus, while Beck's Cognitive Model of Depression presents another reason for the inability to enjoy reinforcement, it lacks – similar to Lewinsohn's hypothesis – considerations of peoples' demographic or individual differences.

It has been demonstrated that Lewinsohn's early behavioural theory was revolutionary for our understanding of the aetiology and symptomology of depression, but overgeneralises the heterogeneity of the disorder. Lewinsohn's work significantly contributed to our understanding of reductions of reinforcement being a reason for the development of depression. He also shed light on reduction of behaviour being a symptom of depression and how this maintains the lack of reinforcement and depression. Thus, he established that antecedents, problem behaviours, and consequences can interact with each other in a self-perpetuating cycle. While his theory contributed to today's knowledge of certain cases of reactive depression, and specific reasons why individuals might be unable to obtain and enjoy reinforcement, it overgeneralises depression. Lewinsohn did not consider the multitude of mediating and moderating factors of depression, and treated the factors he *did* describe – pleasant activities, social skills, and social anxiety - as homogenous constructs, overlooking their own complexities.

It has been demonstrated that some alternative psychological theories of depression align with Lewinsohn's theories, while others show differences to it. While an extensive review of alternative theories was not within the scope of this paper, the alternative theories we did look at served as critical assessments for Lewinsohn's theory. Furthermore, the wide range of complexities of the aetiology and symptomology of depression – as well as the many depressive disorders sub-categorical to clinical depression could not be explored in depth. This however emphasises that "depression is a highly complex disorder influenced by multiple factors, and it is clear that no single theory can fully explain its aetiology and persistence" (Bernaras, Jaureguizar, & Garaigordobil, 2019, p.6).

Bibliography

Abreu, P. R., & Santos, C. E. (2008). Behavioral models of depression: a critique of the emphasis on positive reinforcement. *International Journal of Behavioral Consultation and Therapy*, 4(2), 130-145.

American Psychiatric Association. (2013). *Diagnostic and statistical manual of mental disorder,* (5th ed.). Arlington, VA: Author.

Andreeva, E., Magusson Hanson, L. L., Westerlund, H., Theorell, T., & Brenner, M. H. (2015). Depressive symptoms as a cause and effect of job loss in men and women: evidence in the context of organisational downsizing from the Swedish Longitudinal Occupational Survey of Health. *BMC Public Health,* 15(1), 1049-1072.

Beck, A. T. (1967). *Depression: Clinical, experimental and theoretical aspects.* New York: Hoeber.

Beck, A. T., & Harrison, R. (1983). Cognitions, attitudes and personality dimensions in depression. *Br. J. Cognitive Psychotherapy,* 1-16.

Beck, A. T., Crain, A. L., Solberg, J., Unützer, J., Glasgow, R. E., Maciosek, M. V., & Whitebird, R. (2011). Severity of depression and magnitude of productivity loss. *Annals of Family Medicine,* 9(4), 305-311. doi: 10.1370/afm.1260

Bernaras, E., Jaureguizar, J., & Garaigordobil, M. (2019). Child and adolescent depression: A review of theories, evaluation instruments, prevetion programs, and treatments. *Frontiers in Psychology,* 10(542), 1-24. doi: 10.3389/fpsy.2019.0054

Bowlby, J. (1969). *Attachment and loss: Attachment.* New York: Basic Books.

Braet, C., Wante, L., Van Beveren, M., & Theuwis, L. (2015). Is the cognitive triad a clear marker of depressive symptoms in youngster? *European Child and Adolescence Psychiatry,* 24, 1261-1268. doi: 10.1007/s00787-015-0674-8

Bubonya, M., Cobb-Clark, D. A., & Wooden, M. (2016). Mental health and productivity at

work: does what you do matter? *Melbourne Institute Working Paper,* 16(6), 86-95.

Clarke, D. M., & Currie, K. C. (2009). Depression, anxiety and their relationship with

chronic disease: A review of the epidemiology, risk and treatment evidence. *Medical*

Journal of Australia, 190, 54-60.

Cole, D. A., Martin, J. M., Powers, B., & Truglio, R. (1996). Modeling causal relations

between academic and social competence and depression: A multitrait-multimethod

longitudinal study of children. *Journal of Abnormal Psychology,* 105, 258-270.

Costello, D. M. (1972). Depression: Loss of reinforcers or loss of reinforcer effectiveness?

Behavior Therapy, 3, 240-247.

Coyne, J. C. (1976). Toward an interactional description of depression. *Psychiatry: Journal*

for the Study of Interpersonal Processes, 39, 28-40.

Daviss, W. B., & Bond, J. B. (2016). Comorbid ADHD and depression: assessment and

treatment strategies. *Psychiatric Times,* 33(9), 24-42.

Dean, J., & Keshavan, M. (2017). The neurobiology of depression: an integrative view. *Asian*

Journal of Psychiatry, 27, 101-111. doi: 10:1016/j.ajp.2017.01.025

Deci, E. L., & Ryan, R. M. (1985). *Intrinsic motivation and self-determination in human*

behavior. New York: Plenum.

Eberhart, N. K., & Hammen, C. L. (2006). Interpersonal predictors of onset of depression

during the transition to adulthood. *Personal Relations,* 13, 195-206.

Fairlie, P. (2013). Meaningful work is healthy work. In R. J. Burke, & C. L. Cooper, *The*

fulfilling workplace: The organization's role in achieving individual and

organizational health (pp. 187-205). Surrey: Gower Publishing.

Fauziyyah, A., & Ampuni, S. (2018). Depression tendencies, social skills, and loneliness among college students in Yogyakarta. *Journal Psikologi, 45*(2), 98-106. doi: 10.22146/jpsi.36324

Hames, J. L., & Jones, T. E. (2013). Interpersonal processes in depression. *Annual Review of Clinical Psychology, 9,* 355-377.

Harris, M. A., & Orth, U. (2019). The link between self-esteem and social relationships: A meta-analysis of longitudinal studies. *Journal of Personality and Social Psychology,* 1-19. doi: http://dx.doi:org/10.1057/pspp0000265

Hirschfeld, M. (2001). The comorbidity of major depression and anxiety disorders: recognition and management in primary care. *Primary Care Companion in Clinical Psychiatry, 3*(6), 244-254.

Ingram, R. E. (1984). Toward an information-processing analysis of depression. *Cognitive Therapy and Research, 8,* 443-478.

Jacobs, L., & Joseph, S. (1997). Cognitive Triad Inventory and its association with symptoms of depression and anxiety in adolescents. *Personality and Individual Differences, 22*(5), 769-770. doi: 10.1007/BF01173284

Kang, H., Kim, S., Bae, K., Kim, S. W., Shin, I., Yoon, J., & Kim, J. (2015). Comorbidity of depression with physical disorders: research and clinical implications. *Chonnam Medical Journal, 51*(8), 8-18. doi: http://dx.doi.org/10.4068/cmj.2015.51.1.8

Kanter, J. W., Busch, A. M., Weeks, C. E., & Landes, S. J. (2008). The nature of clinical depression: symptoms, syndromes, and behavioural analysis. *The Behavioral Analyst, 31*(4), 1-21.

Lewinsohn, P. M. (1974). A behavioural approach to depression. In R. J. Friedman, & M. M. Katz, *The psychology of depression: Contemporary theory and research* (pp. 157-185). New York: Wiley.

Lewinsohn, P. M. (1974). Clinical and theoretical aspects of depression. In K. S. Calhoun, H.

E. Adams, & K. M. Mitchel, *Innocative Treatment Methods in Psychopathology* (pp.

63-120). New York: Wiley.

Lewinsohn, P. M., & Graf, M. (1973). Pleasant activites and depression. *Journal of*

Consulting and Clinical Psychology, 41(2), 261-268.

Li, S., Tan, J., & Liu, X. (2008). Continual training of attentional bias in social anxiety.

Behavioral Research and Therapy, 46(8), 905-912. doi: 10.1016/j.brat.2008.04.005

Makkar, S. R., & Griham, J. R. (2011). Social anxiety and the effects of negative self-

imagery on emotion, cognition, and post-event processing. *Behavioral Research and*

Therapy, 49(10), 654-664. doi: 10.1016/j.brat.2011.07.004

Natale, M. (1977a). Effects of induced elation-depression on speech in the initial interview.

Journal of Consulting and Clinical Psychology, 45, 45-52.

Natale, M. (1977b). Induction of mood states and their effect on gaze behaviors. *Journal of*

Consulting and Clinical Psychology, 45, 960.

Navarro-Abal, Y., Climent-Rodríguez, J. A., López-López, M. J., & Gómez-Salgado, J.

(2018). Psychological coping with job loss. Empirical study to contribute to the

development of unemployed people. *International Journal of Environmental*

Research and Public Health, 1787(15), 1-11. doi: 10.3390/ijerph15081787

Pössel, P. (2009). Cognitive Triad Inventiory (CTI): Psychometric properties and factor

structure of the German translation. *Journal of Behavior Therapy and Experimental*

Psychiatry, 40(2), 240-247. doi: http://dx.doi.org/10.1016/j.jbtep.2008.12.001

Rehm, L. (2015). *Cognitive and behavioral theories of depression.* New York: John Wiley &

Sons.

Rodebaugh, T. L., Lim, M. H., Fernandez, K. C., Langer, J. K., Weisman, J. S., Tonge, N., . .

. Shumaker, E. A. (2014). Self and friend's differing views of social anxiety disorders' effects on friendship. *Journal of Abnormal Psychology,* 123(4), 715-724.

doi: https://doi.org/10.1037/abn0000015

Schneier, F. R., Johnsohn, J., Hornig, C. D., Liebowitz, W. R., & Weissman, M. M. (1992).

Social phobia. Comorbidity and morbidity in an epidemiologic sample. *Archives of*

General Psychiatry, 49(4), 282-288. doi: 10.1001/archpsyc.1992.01820040034004

Segrin, C. (1993). Social skills deficits and psychosocial problems: antecedent, concomitant,

or consequence? *Journal of Social and Clinical Psychology,* 12, 336-353.

Segrin, C. (1996). The relationship between social skills deficits and psychosocial problems:

A test of a vulnerability model. *Communcation Research,* 23, 425-450.

Segrin, C. (2000). Social skills deficits associated with depression. *Clinical Psychology*

Review, 20(3), 379-403.

Skinner, B. F. (1953). *Sience and human behavior.* Oxford: Macmillan.

Stein, M. B., Fuetsch, M., Höfler, M., Lieb, R., & Wittchen, H. U. (2001). Social anxiety

disorder and the risk of depression: a prospective community study of adolescents and

young adults. *Archives of General Psychiatry,* 58(3), 251-256.

Stolove, C. A., Galatzer-Levy, I. R., & Bonanno, G. A. (2017). Emergence of depression

following job loss propectively predicts lower rates of reemployment. *Psychiatry*

Research, 253(1), 79-83.

Stopa, L., Brown, M. A., & Hirsch, C. R. (2012). The effects of repreated imagery practice

on self-concept, anxiety and performance in socially anxious participants. *Journal of*

Experimental Psychopathology, 3(2), 223-242. doi: 10.5127/jep.021511

Weinstein, S. M., & Mermelstein, R. (2007). Relations between daily activites and adolescent

mood: The role of autonomy. *Journal of Clinical Child and Adolesence Psychology,*

36(2), 182-194.

Wierzbicki, M. (1984). Social skills deficits and subsequent depressed mood in students. *Personality and Social Psychology Bulletin,* 10, 605-610.

Wierzbicki, M., & McCabe, M. (1988). Social skills and subsequent depressive symtomatology in children. *Journal of Clinical Child Psychology,* 3, 203-208.

World Health Organisation. (30. January 2020). *Depression.* Retrieved from World health Organization: https://www.who.int/news-room/fact-sheets/detail/depression

YOUR KNOWLEDGE HAS VALUE

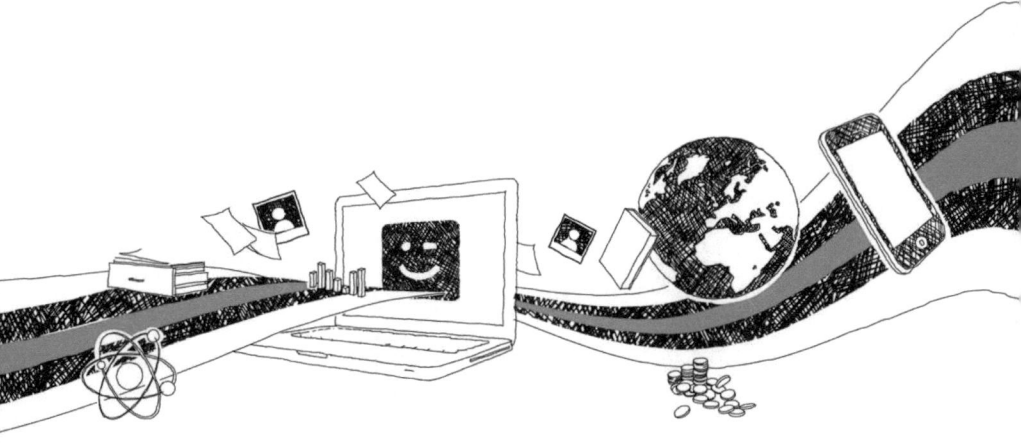

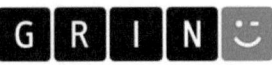